Yoga Beyond the Poses
AYURVEDA

*The Ultimate Beginner's Guide
to Discover the basics of Ayurveda!*

Shreyanada Natha

Illustrator
Mattias Långström

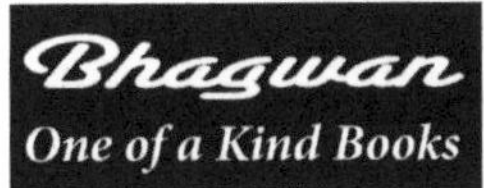

Yoga Beyond the Poses
Ayurveda

*The Ultimate Beginner's Guide
to Discover the basics of Ayurveda!*

Shreyanada Natha

ISBN 9789198839265

✳ ✳ ✳

2 FREE PREMIUM BONUS!

*#1. Download the **AUDIOBOOK** at the back of the book!*

*#2. Download **CHAKRA-INDEX IN COLOR** here!*

SCAN QR-CODE or go to:

https://bit.ly/47wdFVZ

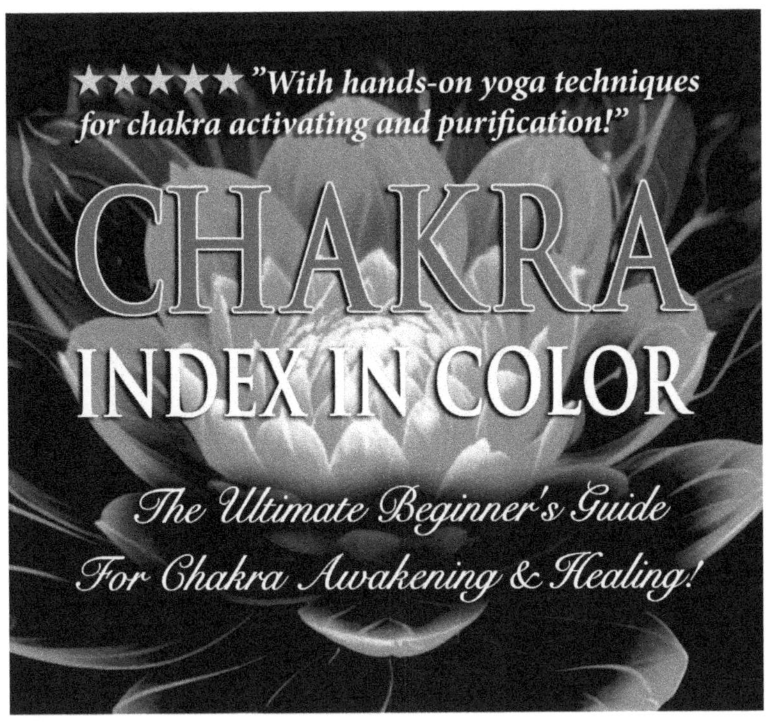

FREE PREMIUM Audiobook
Authentic Yoga Nidra Meditation – Vishuddhi Chakra Awakening!

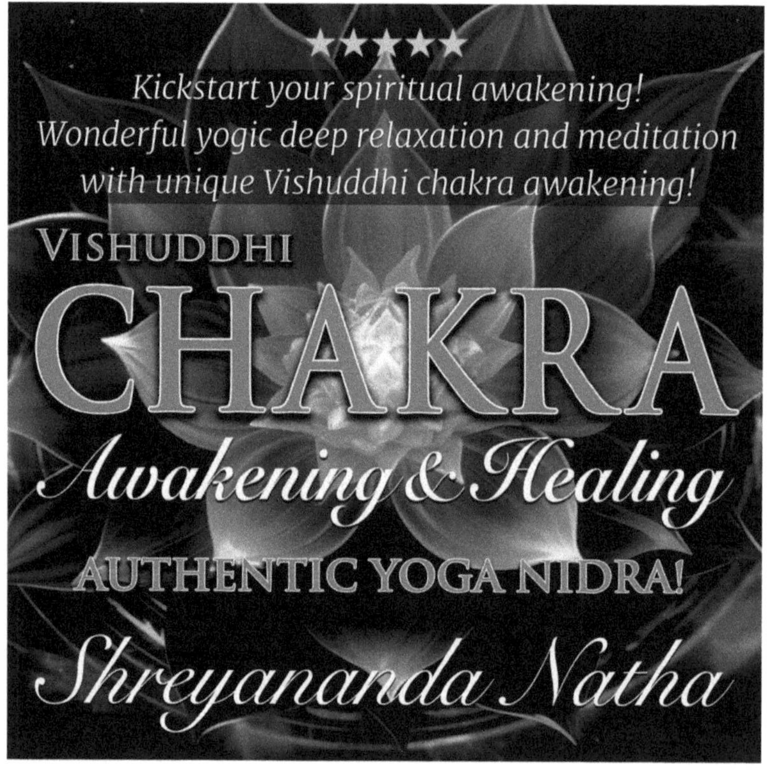

*Download the **AUDIOBOOK** at the back of the book!*

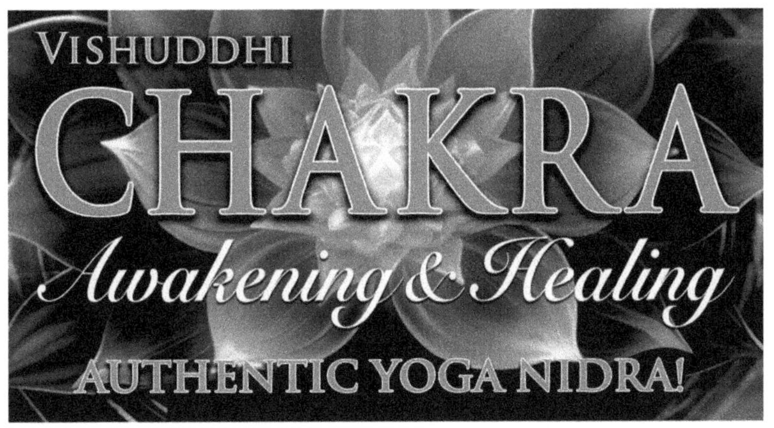

Kickstart your spiritual awakening! Wonderful yogic deep relaxation and meditation with unique Vishuddhi chakra awakening and healing.

PRESENTATION

Yoga Nidra, or yogic sleep, is a unique meditation process that's powerfully profound and healing for body, mind, and spirit.

Practitioners are led into a state of deep relaxation and the experience of our chakra system.

Yoga Nidra offers extensive benefits, yet it is one of the most straightforward yoga practices.

All you have to do is put on your most comfortable clothes, find a quiet space, lie down on your back, and play the meditation.

Yoga Beyond the Poses – Ayurveda
The Ultimate Beginner's Guide to Discover the basics of Ayurveda!
Including A Premium Audiobook: Yoga Nidra Meditation – Vishuddhi Chakra Awakening And Healing!

The book describes the basics of Ayurveda. Learn how to use yoga, breathing exercises, and meditation for different doshas (personality types), how to practice oil massage at home, how to practice pulse diagnosis, and much more. It penetrates deeply but remains easy to read, educational, and understandable. A must on the bookshelf for anyone interested in Ayurveda and who quickly wants to know more.

The book is part of a series of seven yoga books, Yoga Beyond the Poses: The Ultimate Beginner's Guide to Yoga, that delve into the seven key areas of yoga.

INCLUDING A PREMIUM AUDIOBOOK: AUTHENTIC YOGA NIDRA MEDITATION – VISHUDDHI CHAKRA AWAKENING & HEALING!
Kickstart your spiritual awakening! Wonderful yogic deep relaxation and meditation with unique Vishuddhi chakra awakening and healing.

Yoga Nidra, or yogic sleep, is a unique meditation process that's powerfully profound and healing for body, mind, and

spirit. Practitioners are led into a state of deep relaxation and the experience of our chakra system. Yoga Nidra offers extensive benefits, yet it is one of the most straightforward yoga practices. All you have to do is put on your most comfortable clothes, find a quiet space, lie down on your back, and play the meditation. –
Download the audiobook at the back of the book!

ABOUT THE BOOK SERIES
YOGA BEYOND THE POSES: *The Ultimate Beginner's Guide to Yoga!*

The book is part of a seven-book yoga series, Yoga Beyond the Poses: The Ultimate Beginner's Guide to Yoga, that delve into yoga's seven most important areas. They are straightforward to read, educational, and fascinating. A must on the bookshelf for anyone interested in yoga who quickly wants to know more.

MY NAME AND MY MISSION

Shreyananda Natha was the name I was given when I was initiated into the Natha Order and received the master mantra – the Shodasi mantra, after studying yoga and tantra for over twelve years, the highest mantra in yoga and tantra. It means "he who knows".

After practicing yoga and meditation continuously for over twenty years, having a yoga school for many years, and le-

THE AUTHOR

*Shreyananda Natha is the author of popular and best-selling
yoga books. He has, among other things, written one of the
most comprehensive books about yoga – EVERYTHING
ABOUT YOGA and the study book – TEACHING YOGA
AND MEDITATION BEYOND THE POSES. He is also a
certified yoga and meditation teacher according to the EYTF
international guidelines. He has undergone multi-year yoga
teacher training under the guidance of Swami Omananda at
Satyananda Ashram and holds the highest initiation in the
tantric Natha order. He frequently travels to Asia and India
to learn and gain knowledge and inspiration. He has immer-
sed himself in tantric rituals and is known for his extensive
knowledge of yoga, deep relaxation, and meditation.*

*"There is no authority that can say what yoga is. When you
surrender yourself completely and fully and experience yoga
without limitations and doubts, the true encounter with yoga
occurs when you become one with the true experience within
you. Only then will you understand what yoga is – for you.
When you are no longer limited by neatness, shyness, and
artificial thought patterns that act as a filter between you
and the transformation. Yoga is a cultural-historical wealth
still passed on from teacher to student and helps man find
his way back to his true nature. It opens us up and attracts
awareness. It strengthens our self-esteem, and our person's
entire spectrum of possibilities suddenly becomes visible.*

Yoga is not difficult or strange. You don't have to become a vegan, a monk, or be able to stand on your head. You just need to do your yoga regularly; the rest will take care of itself. You can use yoga and meditation to feel better, both physically and mentally, but also to achieve success and develop in all areas of life – here and now."

Good luck!

NAMASTÉ

I want to thank the teachers and students I've had over the years who have made my journey with yoga so enjoyable. Thank you for all the inspiration you have given me and for making this book possible. The yoga masters who no longer live among us – live on with each new person who immerses themselves in the yoga tradition.

Sri Swami Sivananda, Sri Swami Satyananda, Sri Tirumalai Krishnamacharya, Sri Swami Vishnudevananda, Sri K. Pattabhi Jois, Osho, Swami Nirdosha, Swami Omananda, Swami Janakananda, Ole Schmidt, Turiya, Maryam Abrishami and Sanna Kuittinen.

People who all searched for answers to what they sensed through an activated Ajna chakra. In yoga, they have learned the principles behind the universe, the collective consciousness, and the creative force, Kundalini Shakti. The duality behind everything, both what we see and what we don't see. Together, we are helped to pass on the previously secret knowledge about our gunas, nadis, and chakras to all who want to become a Rishi.

Aum Shri Durgayai Namaha

Shreyananda Natha

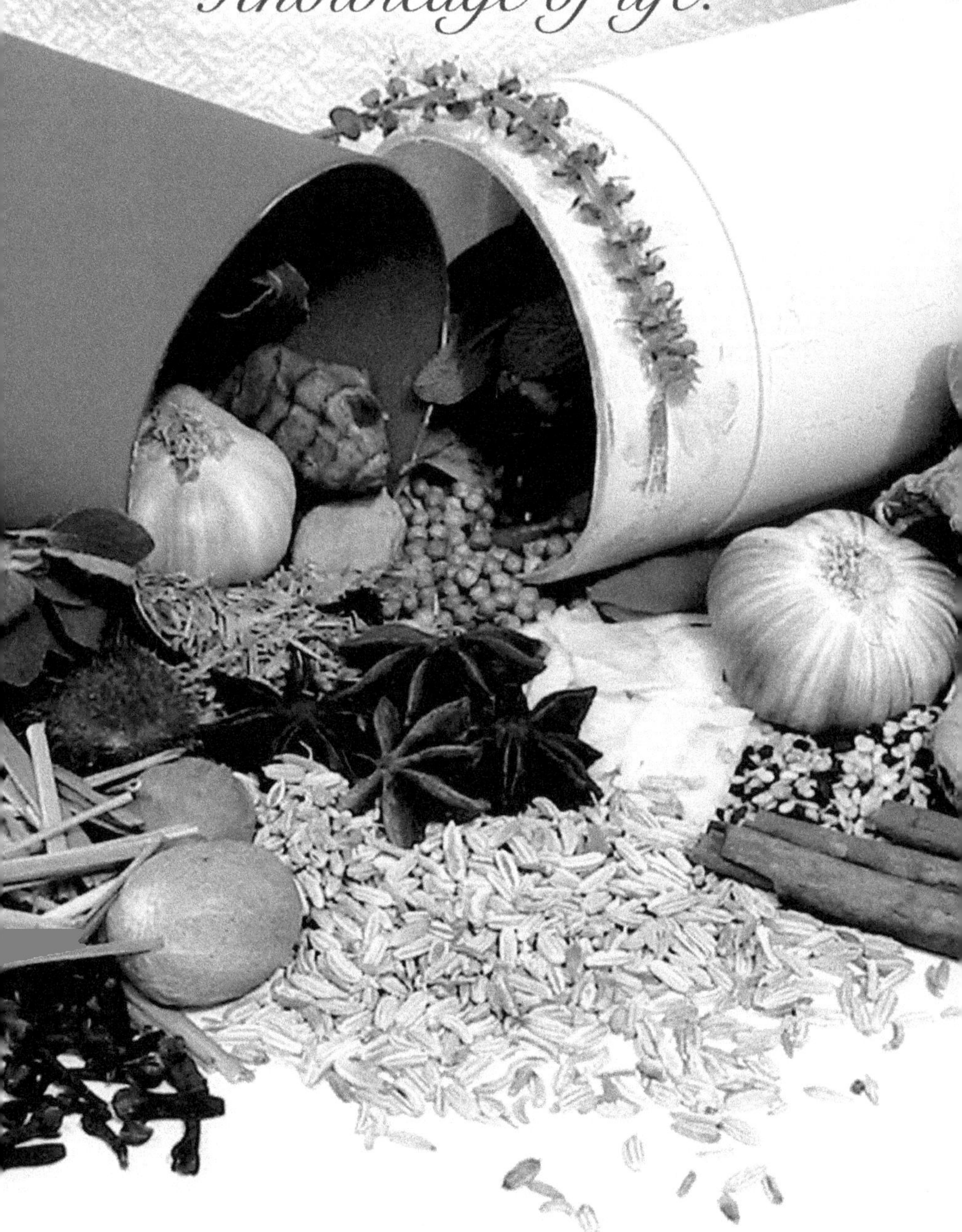
AYURVEDA
Knowledge of life!

ॐ

AYURVEDA

VATA, PITTA & KAPHA

Ayurveda is an Indian health science with roots in the Vedic tradition. Both yoga and Ayurveda originally came into being as Vedic teachings and are believed to be more than five thousand years old.

Ayur means life, and Veda means knowledge – the knowledge/science about life. With the help of Ayurveda, we can learn to live in balance with our life force and our entire divine consciousness.

In Ayurveda, the whole person is treated, not just the sick. When you create balance, you simultaneously release the self-healing forces. Ayurveda develops the health potential we have within us and, at the same time, expands our consciousness.

Ayurveda and yoga originate from the same tradition and have been practiced together for thousands of years. It is often forgotten, resulting in yoga and Ayurveda being taught separately. Both classical yoga and Ayurveda take the whole person into account physically, mentally, and spiritually.

You could say that Ayurveda is a tradition of Vedic knowledge that describes how to heal the body and mind, while yoga is a tradition of Vedic knowledge that describes the path to self-insight. Achieving self-insight requires that the body and mind are in balance.

UPAVEDAS

Ayurveda is part of the four upavedas that supplement the four Vedas.

Ayurveda is also closely related to the practice of Veda as it treats various mantras and methods to cure diseases.

The four upavedas are:

1. Ayurveda – knowledge of life.

2. Gandharva veda – knowledge of culture, art and music's role in spiritual development. For example, there is music for various disease conditions.

3. Dhanur veda – knowledge of the importance of behavior for spiritual development.

4. Sthapatya veda – knowledge of the importance of architecture for spiritual development. This veda is also known as vastu and is reminiscent of feng shui. Feng Shui is a philosophy that practices arranging building structures and objects within living spaces to create balance and energy.

THREE DOSHAS

In Ayurveda, three doshas or energy principles control all life processes internally and externally. Our biological existence is based on the interplay between these three energy principles. Doshas combines the five elements: space, air, fire, water, and earth.

The doshas also determine what personality type you are. It is usually said that you have one or two doshas that dominate. According to astrology, the influence of the celestial bodies (grahas) during conception determines which dosha becomes the most dominant in each person. There is dosha type one, dosha type two, and dosha type three.

In our yoga practice, it is essential to understand how the doshas affect us. Knowing the energy principles and how they act and interact in and around us, we can take full advantage of fine yogic techniques to create balance and harmony in our physical and subtle bodies. We can adapt our yoga practice to the needs and personality types that we need to achieve the best possible results.

In Ayurveda, yoga is used to maintain a healthy lifestyle and as a treatment method for diseases. Asanas, pranayamas, and meditation are among the best methods to maintain balance in the doshas.

VATA	**PITTA**	**KAPHA**
Space / air.	*Fire / water.*	*Water / soil.*
Movement.	*Combustion.*	*Structure.*
Dry.	*A little oily.*	*Fat/oily.*
Light.	*Light.*	*Heavy.*
Cold.	*Warm/hot.*	*Cold.*
Very fast.	*Fast.*	*Slow.*
Hearing / feeling.	*The eyes.*	*Taste / smell.*
The moon.	*The sun.*	*Earth.*

Vata is kinetic energy in various ways and the force that allows the other two doshas to move. Vata exists as air in our organs, joints, and bones. On a deeper level, vata is the life force within us and the power of thought that moves in our minds. Vata controls the central nervous system, the movements of the heart, the intestines, the lungs, the thought processes, and the communication between the mind and the body.

Pitta is responsible for the metabolism and conversion process in the body. In addition to digestion, it melts our impressions of the outside world, emotions, and ideas. Pitta provides us with intelligence, courage, and vitality. With pitta, we gain motivation and sight to reach our goals in life. You can see pitta in photosynthesis, which is nature's combustion.

Kapha is the one who unites. The stable structure is associated with bone structure, mucous membranes, joints, rocks, and mountains. Kapha provides us with emotions and feelings that contribute to love, care, devotion, and faith, which causes us to maintain harmony within ourselves and unite with others.

Vata, pitta, and kapha are closely linked and always work together. In every single cell in the body, these three interact. For vata to be in balance, pitta and kapha must exist in the right proportion because they have these elements in the form of water and fire. Vata is the easiest to get out of balance but also the easiest to rebalance. Pitta, in turn, needs to be watered with vata's properties of movement and decomposition (start the fire / dampen the fire) and also kapha's building and preserving properties to keep the fire alive. Kapha needs vata to start the movement and pitta for its stimulus and warming properties. Consequently, we see that none of the doshas can exist without the other; they are all equally important.

RAJAS, TAMAS & SATTVA

Prakriti consists of three varying qualities: rajas, tamas, and sattva. Rajas is the active, stimulating, and positive force contributing to change. Tamas is the passive and harmful force that keeps the old. Sattva is the neutral and balancing force that harmonizes the positive and the negative. All three energies are necessary for everything that happens, even on the spiritual plane.

Sattva is the light, the love, and the life. It is the higher spiritual power that makes us develop our consciousness. Rajas is the passion, the twilight, and what changes. It is the vital force that lacks stability. It gives rise to emotional fluctuations such as fear and desire, love and hate. Tamas is the dark, the insensitive, and the dead. The lower material force pulls us to unconsciousness, stagnation, listlessness, and heaviness. Unmanifested Prakriti keeps these three in balance. Rajas and tamas get sattva together. When Prakriti is manifested, these qualities are distinguished.

Sattva gives rise to the mind, rajas generates the life force, and tamas stands for form and substance as the physical body. Yoga and Ayurveda want to develop the sattvic state. In yoga, sattva is the higher quality that makes us grow spiritually. In Ayurveda, sattva is the state of balance in which the healing property is released.

YOGIC AND AYURVEDIC DIET

In Ayurveda, diet plays a considerable role and lays the foundation for all other therapeutic approaches and healing processes. Without a proper and balanced diet, other medicines have no significant effect. The food is used as medicine. A sattvic diet is advocated because sattva creates balance. A sattvic diet is traditionally based on ahimsa, an ethical principle of not causing harm to other living beings. As far as possible, the food should have grown naturally in a harmonious environment as such food carries a lot of prana and pure awareness.

Yogis worldwide are usually very aware of what they eat, but a traditional yogic diet and an Ayurvedic one are different. Ayurveda wants to create balance and build good physical health. In yoga, you want to develop and change body awareness. In short, Ayurveda wants to make physical health, and yoga helps us get beyond the body's limits. Many traditional yogic paths are ascetic, where solid, simple raw foods with detoxifying effects are common. However, these have a water-raising impact. A Standard Ayurvedic diet is instead based on well-cooked and nutritious food to strengthen us physically and prevent doshas from becoming unbalanced or unnecessarily wet.

A traditional yogic diet increases the elements of space / ether and air (vata) to detoxify and open up the mind. The-

refore, raw food and fasting are recommended. By reducing the body, you expand the mind. Another significant factor in the yogic diet is prana. A raw diet is rich in prana. By following a raw diet, you increase the flow of prana in the body and thus purify nadis. Breathing exercises improve the digestive fire in the body, allowing the food to be digested even though it's not cooked.

However, only some of us can digest this type of food satis-factorily. It is especially true for vata people with varying digestive fire, but even kapha and pitta can have difficulty with this. Therefore, most non-ascetics feel better from a well-cooked, warm diet that is easy to digest.

An Ayurvedic diet is not necessarily sattvic but focuses more on creating physical health. On the other hand, a Yogic diet places the most significant emphasis on the food's satiety, which can increase a dosha. You can choose sattvic food adapted to your dominant dosha type for an optimal diet. Sattvic food includes dairy products, natural oils, herbal teas, sweet spices, fruits, fresh juices, vegetables, cereals, legumes, nuts, seeds, and honey. For a sattvic diet, eating the correct type of food at the right time during the day is divided into vata, pitta, and kapha time. In Ayurveda, it is recommended to eat light food for breakfast because Kapha time prevails, and heavy food also weighs down the mind and body. The biggest goal should be to eat in the middle of

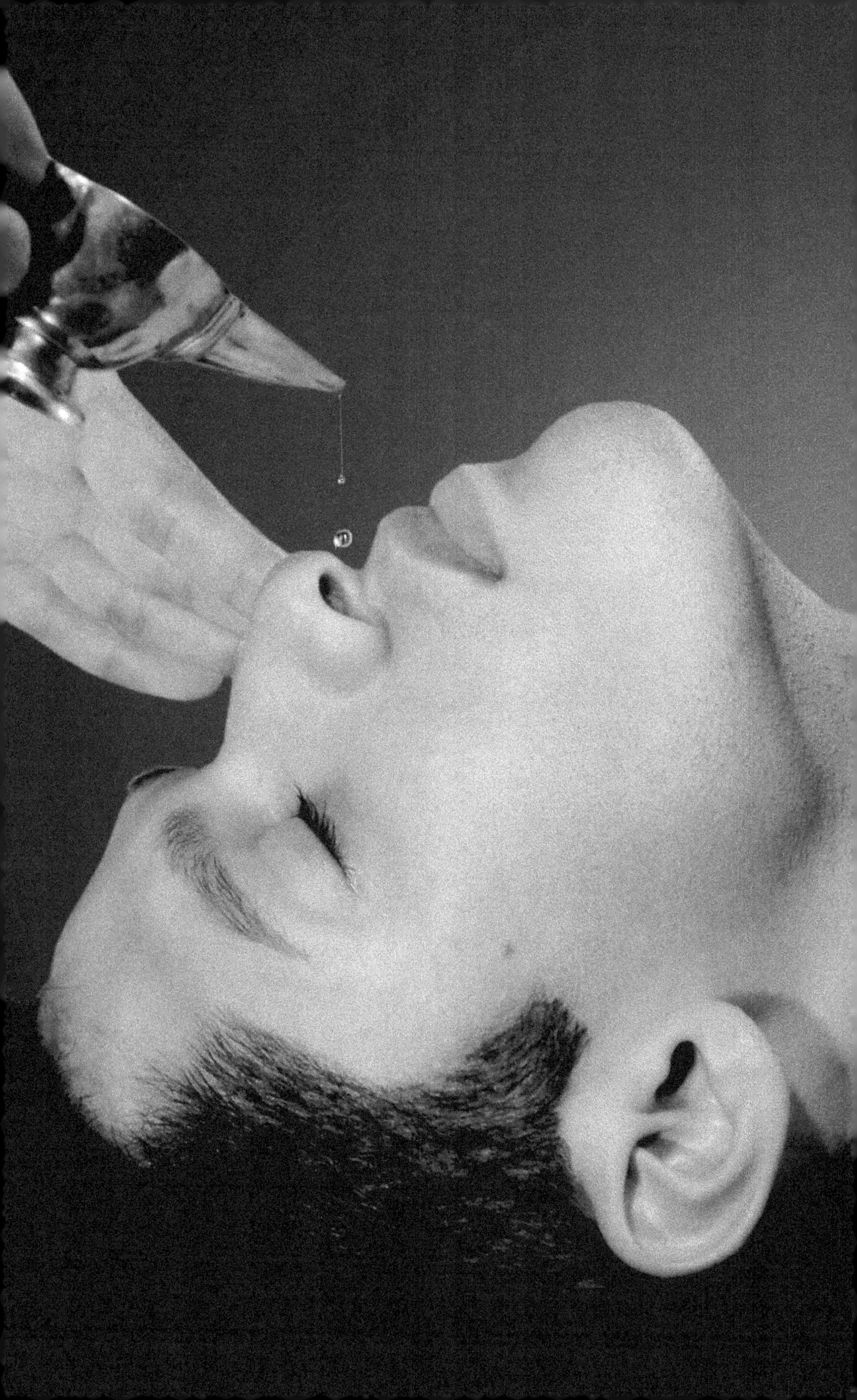

the day during pitta time when digestion is at its strongest. In the evening, you should not eat heavy foods or too close to bedtime as it disturbs both sleep and the natural cleansing of waste materials.

THE SIX TASTES
Six different flavors affect each dosha in different ways. Each flavor consists of a combination of two elements.

Sweet – water and soil.
Balances vata and pitta. It increases kapha—for example, vegetables, oils, milk and rice.

Sour – fire and soil.
Balances vata. It increases pitta and kapha—for example, citrus, yogurt, cheese, and vinegar.

Salt – fire and water.
Balances vata. It increases pitta and kapha—for example, seaweed, tamari, and table salt.

Pungent – fire and air.
It decreases kapha. It increases pitta and vata—for example, strong spices such as pepper, onion, and ginger.

Bitter – space and air.
Balances pitta and kapha. It increases vata—for example, green leafy vegetables and turmeric.

Astringent – air and soil.

Balances pitta and kapha. It increases vata—for example, beans, lentils, and unripe bananas.

TIP

Try to eat in silence and in a relaxed manner. Focus on the meal and not on anything else at the same time. Eat foods you like and avoid cold foods. Avoid eating when you feel anxious, angry, or sad. Drink boiled water with food, not milk. Eat freshly prepared food as much as possible and avoid leftovers, as the nutrients have already been lost. The food must be equipped with love and awareness.

AGNI

In Ayurveda, the body's digestive fire – agni, is significant. If the fire is too weak, the food cannot be digested satisfactorily, and nutrients are lost. The food we eat then becomes ama (slag products), which strains our bodies. In Ayurveda, a weak digestive fire is the root cause of most diseases. Our modern life and our stress are major contributing factors to poor digestion. We tend to gulp down food instead of enjoying it.

When we have a balance between the doshas, the agni will also be in balance. A sign of this is when we regularly feel a healthy appetite.

The agni is weakened when we overeat, snack, or eat even though we are not hungry. Refrigerated food, prolonged fasting, and poorly chewed food are also contributing factors.

When vata is increased, digestion becomes irregular. It can change from fast to slow; sometimes, you can feel an intense hunger. Stomach problems are also part of the picture.

When pitta gets out of balance, the agni becomes too strong. You may experience extreme hunger, often shortly after eating. It contributes to nutrients not being absorbed by the body, and in the long run, you can suffer from stomach ulcers.

When kapha is elevated, digestion becomes very slow instead. You experience a heavy feeling after eating, and feelings of hunger are weak.

AGNI YOGA

Both yoga and Ayurveda carry the knowledge of the divine fire, the agni. We learn to control the fire to create balance and to develop. The cosmic fire exists everywhere, in ourselves and around us. In the body, we see the agni in the form of our digestive fire; on a finer level, the agni corresponds to our eternal consciousness. Without fire, our development and evolution will stop.

In Ayurveda, we learn to balance the function of the agni physically by taking care of our digestive fire, which then lays the foundation for good health.

In yoga, the focus is on the pranic agni and the fire of meditation, which are essential for our enlightenment. Various fire rituals are performed every day in yoga traditions. Still, we may be most familiar with the Breath of Fire exercise, which cleanses the body's energy channels and increases the flow of prana in the body.

YOGA'S IMPACT ON OUR THREE DOSHAS

ASANAS AND AYURVEDA

Asanas release tension and energy blockages that may have occurred, thereby keeping the body's tissues, joints, and organs in the best possible shape. The positions stretch and strengthen the muscles, and the spine is kept flexible, making it possible for the energy to flow freely through nerves that belong to our organs and glands. Our tissues are, therefore, cleansed systematically, preparing the body for more advanced yogic exercises.

Asanas prepare you for breathing exercises and meditation. They not only have a physical purpose, but they also affect us on a practical, mental, and spiritual level. From the beginning, asanas have aimed to counter rajas, the turbulent energy within us that distracts the mind.

Asanas help to balance and release the prana in the body, which prepares us for breathing exercises. Our senses are turned inward, which facilitates mind control (pratyahara). When our thoughts are still, the mind is calmed so that we can concentrate (dharana) and meditate (dhyana).

Diet and asanas are the two most essential factors in creating good health and counteracting imbalances and diseases in the long run.

Spices, herbs, and various breathing exercises are used to balance the prana in the body. A proper posture and diet are required as a basis to enable this. Our posture is of great importance for our health and consciousness. The body and the mind influence each other through subtle channels in the body through which foods and our thoughts flow. The musculoskeletal system holds the channels together, the shape of which is determined by our posture. Improper posture causes stress in the body and blocks these channels. The energy cannot flow optimally, and residual products and toxins have a chance to accumulate. It eventually leads to discomfort in the body, pain, and illness.

It is easy for asanas to become the mainstay of yoga practice. If you want to participate in yoga on a deeper level, give equal time to asanas, pranayamas, and meditation. An exaggerated and unconscious execution of asanas leads to a fixation on the body and boosts our physical ego: this leads to a rigid and undeveloped mind and emotions. Never exaggerate the exercises or force the body into a position that will cause more tension and injury.

ASANAS AND OUR AGE
Infants and children are by nature soft and flexible in the

body. Practicing asanas early means maintaining the softness and correct posture for life.

Vinyasas are suitable for younger people because many rajas prevail in body and mind, and they need vinyasas to mature. After twenty-four, one should move on to inner yoga and develop the mind by studying yogic texts.

After forty-eight, the mind develops at the same speed as the physical energies are withdrawn. It would help if you meditate more, but asanas are still crucial for keeping the body supple and healthy.

At sixty–five, the vata age, the body fluids slowly decrease and dry out. The body becomes stiffer, and joint diseases are common. With the help of asanas, you can keep your body in shape and balance excess vata.

At the age of seventy-two, the mind develops even more. It is the time for deep meditation. Asanas continue to be essential to slow down aging.

ASANAS FOR VATA

Vata people often have a slim and thin physique. They are very flexible and mobile when young but quickly develop stiffness as they age. Vatas often suffer from joint problems in middle age. They are often cold, have dry skin, cracked joints, and poor blood circulation. Vata people are naturally nervous and scared, which makes them tense in their shoulders and back. Asanas are essential for vata people, for both their health and their ability to meditate. Vatas must exercise caution when practicing asanas as they are prone to injury. Soft, flowing exercises at a reasonable speed are preferred.

Mental preparation is essential for vatas: a moment of rest and deep breathing before asanas is necessary. During practice, vatas should start slowly so the circulation awakens and the joints can warm up. Vatas should not be too sweaty as they dry out quickly. Intake of fluid is essential. Asanas should mainly affect the area around the hips and intestines, which is the main seat of vata. Releasing tension from the hips and lumbar spine is essential. Too much stretching and movement can cause over-stretching and weakness.

Sitting positions such as padmasana and vajrasana are good for vata. These have a calming, grounding effect and control apana vayu.

Keeping the spine flexible is essential for vatas, who often accumulate tension here. Exercises that rotate the spine in each direction are good. Matsyendrasana is an example of a pose that releases vata from the nervous system. It is essential to have proper breathing when performing spinal rotation. Otherwise, the pose will have the opposite effect and increase vata.

Forward bending positions have a calming effect and release vata from the back. Combining forward-turning positions with backward-bending positions is essential to maximize the benefits. However, this should be done slowly and carefully. Doing backward bending positions too quickly can stimulate the sympathetic nervous system and our "fight or flight" mechanism. With caution, asanas such as the cobra and the grasshopper have a grounding and strengthening effect on vatas.

Standing poses are perfect for vata. They build strength, give peace, and increase stability.

Vatas should avoid becoming too exhausted. Dynamic asanas should be accompanied by sitting positions, pranayamas, and meditation.

After asanas, vatas should lie and rest in shavasana. It is an optimal time to meditate, with the mind calm and the emotions stable.

Seated poses:
Siddhasana/siddha yoni asana (perfect pose), vajrasana (diamond pose) and simhasana (lion pose).

The sun salutation:
Slowly and consciously.

Standing poses:
Vrksasana (tree pose), trikonasana (triangle pose), virabhadrasana (warrior pose), parighasana (gate pose), and all standing forward bending positions.

Inverted poses:
Shirshasana (headstand), vipareeta karani asana (half shoulder stand).

Backbends:
Bhujangasana (cobra) and shalabhasana (grasshopper).

Forward bends:
All. Especially janu sirsasana (half-butterfly) and pachimottasana (pliers).

Spinal twists:
Lying positions, bharadvajasana (half turn) and shava udarakarshanasana (universal position).

Other:
Shashankasana (hare), parivrtta janu sirsasana (one-legged forward bend in a seated position), navasana (boat), yoga mudra.

Shavasana:
At least twenty minutes.

ASANAS FOR PITTA

Pittas have a medium-sized physique. They often have good muscles and flexibility. Circulation and joint mobility are usually good due to the slightly oily nature of pittas. Pittas usually handle asanas very well, but if overdone, it may lead to hypermobility and stiffness in joints.

Mentally, pitta people are aggressive and like to shine in everything they do. Pittas must be careful about "performing" when it comes to asanas. They can often become perfect at technical but need to remember the spiritual part. Pittas often need to be more ambitious, annoyed, and very driven. Asanas should be used to cool pittas down physically and mentally, helping them turn their intelligence inward to understand themselves better.

Calm breathing and sitting still after powerful asanas are essential to counteract stress. Pittas should avoid overly strenuous exercise and not get too hot. Powerful asanas are ok as long as pittas compensate by using cooling asanas and pranayamas to cool the mind and body towards the end.

Around the navel, heat is created and distributed throughout the body. We have a cooling function in the palate, where saliva is secreted. The heat from the umbilical region moves upwards to reduce the cold produced in the soft palate. The cooling property is protected from heat by standing in a shoulder position or entering the plow position. These positions reverse the positions of the sun and the moon in the body, which creates balance, especially in pitta people. Spinal twists such as matsyendrasana are also suitable for protecting the cooling property without lowering the fire in the body. Positions that release tension and affect the abdominal tract, small intestine, and liver are also beneficial for pittas because pittas accumulate in these areas. The bow, cobra, boat, and fish poses are good. Headstand increases pitta and should be avoided if you do not know how to balance the heat afterward.

Forward bending positions are generally suitable for pittas because they increase the energy around the abdomen and have a cooling and grounding effect. Back-bending positions create more heat and should, therefore, be practiced in moderation and followed by cooling asanas. Seated spinal twists help cleanse the liver and detoxify the pitta.

After asanas, pitta should feel calm, cool, and relaxed in the stomach. The mind should be in a meditative state and not too sharp.

Seated poses:
Most are beneficial except simhasana (the lion), which should be avoided.

The moon greeting:
Cooling for pitta.

Standing poses:
Vrksasana (tree pose), trikonasana (triangle pose), ardha chandrasana (crescent pose).

Standing poses (legs wide apart):
Moordhasana (head on the floor from standing with legs apart), padottanasana (leg lift).

Forward bends:
All seated forward bends are good, especially pada prasar paschimottanasana (forward bend with legs split), kurmasana (turtle) and paschimottanasana (pliers).

Twists:
Ardha matsyendrasana (half spinal rotation).

Other:
Sarvangasana (shoulder stand), vipareeta karani (half shoulder stand), navasana (boat), ardha matsyendrasana (seated spine twisting), bhujangasana (cobra), yoga mudra.

Shavasana:
Medium, long.

ASANAS FOR KAPHA

Kapha types are heavily built and gain weight quickly. They are often inflexible and should not try to push the body into a position like a lotus position, which carries a risk of injury. Kapha's body and joints often do not support these positions. Kaphas must accept how they are built and not try to become thin, slim yogis because their body is not made that way.

Kapha women can be thin when young but gain weight over the years, especially after giving birth. It can weigh down kaphas as they may have difficulty accepting this. In this case, they are expected to use different ways to try to lose weight, such as yoga, although it rarely results. Kaphas must instead work on their attitude toward their body and accept what is natural for them. Kaphas still needs to try to maintain average body weight without starving themselves.

Obesity in kapha is mainly seen on the abdomen and thighs, causing various problems with posture. Increased kapha also causes mucus formation around the breasts and lungs, spreading to different parts of the body and causes duct blockages. These blockages contribute to increased fat accumulation around joints and tissues.

Kapha people are rarely physically active, although needing it to stimulate their metabolism and increase circulation. As kaphas are easily affected by high cholesterol and heart disease, they should exercise cautiously and be mindful not to overwork while still challenging themselves.

As heat triggers the flow in kaphas, exercises that increase heat and make the body sweat are good. Kaphas needs to be pushed to do strenuous exercises that they do not think they can do.

Sitting asanas increase kapha. Pranayamas that increase heat are beneficial before meditation.

Vinyasas such as the sun salutation are good to start the flow. Backward bending positions are also good as they open up the chest, which is the area for kapha. Backbends also increase circulation in the head, which counteracts inertia. Forward bending positions should generally be avoided by kaphas unless they need to calm the nervous system.

Kaphas often suffer from slow digestion. Therefore, exercises like the arch that initiates the flow at the navel region are excellent. The plow is one of the best positions to open up the lungs. Pranayamas create the flow in both body and mind.

After asanas, kaphas should feel light and warm and have increased circulation in the body. The chest and lungs should be open, and the mind should feel clear and alert.

Seated poses:
Simhasana (the lion) and in combination with pranayamas.

The sun salutation:
At a fast pace.

Standing poses:
Virabhadrasana (warrior), Utthita hasta padangusthasana (hand-to-toe stand), bakasana (crow), ardha chandrasana (crescent position).

Inverted poses:
Adho mukha vrksasana (downward facing dog), sirsasana (headstand), sarvangasana (shoulder stand).

Backbends:
Ustrasana (camel pose), shalabasana (grasshopper pose).

Other:
Shava udarakarshanasana (spinal rotation), ardha matsy-endrasana (half spinal rotation), parvatasana (mountain pose), and halasana (plow pose).

Shavasana:
Short.

PRANAYAMAS

Yoga teaches us how to master prana and thus gain access to its more profound powers. When we learn that, we no longer need external pleasure. In this way, we take control of our mind and can heal it and our body. A knowledgeable Ayurveda doctor knows how to redirect the prana in the body to heal the patient. In the same way, food, herbs, and other healing methods influence the prana.

Pranayama is one of the most central exercises in yoga and is the fourth step in classical yoga. The prana cleanses and revitalizes the body before meditation.

With breathing exercises, you slow down and prolong your breath. It causes the life energy – the prana, to manifest itself.

Breathing exercises have a good effect on diseases that affect the respiratory organs, circulation, and nervous system, as well as fatigue and a weak immune system. The whole body is affected by the exercises by massaging the internal organs. The circulation increases in the internal organs and is detoxified. Pranayamas also have an excellent effect on depression, stress, and tension.

PRANA AND APANA

The apana associated with gravity moves downwards and results in disease, aging, death, and unconsciousness. Pra-

na, related to the elements of air and space, moves upwards through our senses. Combining these two energies can strengthen our energy and awaken our higher abilities. Yogic exercises involve redirecting the apana upwards to meet the prana and pulling the prana down to meet the apana. It takes place at the solar plexus, which is the seat of the prana.

Prana – inhalation.
Samana – hold your breath / contract.
Vyana – hold your breath / expand.
Udana – exhale / squeeze out.
Apana – exhale / elimination.

PRANAYAMA AND PRANA AGNI

Pranayamas develop the fire of prana, which is responsible for the body's combustion. It is done by holding your breath. Oxygen acts as food for pranaagni. The carbon dioxide that accompanies the exhalation is its residual product. Holding our breath cleanses our subtle body in the same way that fasting cleanses our physical. Prana agni gives power to Kundalini so it can continue its journey upwards and take with it prana and apana.

PRANAYAMAS AND DOSHAS

Pranayamas affect all doshas. Done correctly, they help balance vata, reduce kapha, and counter pitta. Inhalation relates to kapha and has a constructive effect. Holding the breath *in links to the pitta and is having a transforming impact. Exhalation relates to vata and has a reducing effect.*

Breathing through the right nostril gives power to the pingala nadi and increases pitta. Breathing through the left nostril gives power to ida nadi and increases kapha. Balanced breathing through both nostrils balances vata.

Kapha increases when you breathe through your mouth, which is generally advised against. However, there are some specific breathing exercises where you apply breathing through the mouth which can help the prana to be retained in the sushumna nadi.

VATA

Breathing through the right nostril is revitalizing for vata. Practice with intent in the morning for about ten to fifteen minutes. Breathing through the left nostril has a calming effect and calms the mind. Practice with purpose in the evening to improve night sleep. Bhastrika can help energize and clarify the mind, but it should be done carefully. End the exercise if dizziness occurs.

PITTA

Cooling pranayamas are best suited for pittas. Breathing through the left nostril is beneficial in the evening and in cases of feeling overheated or irritated. Shitali and sitkari

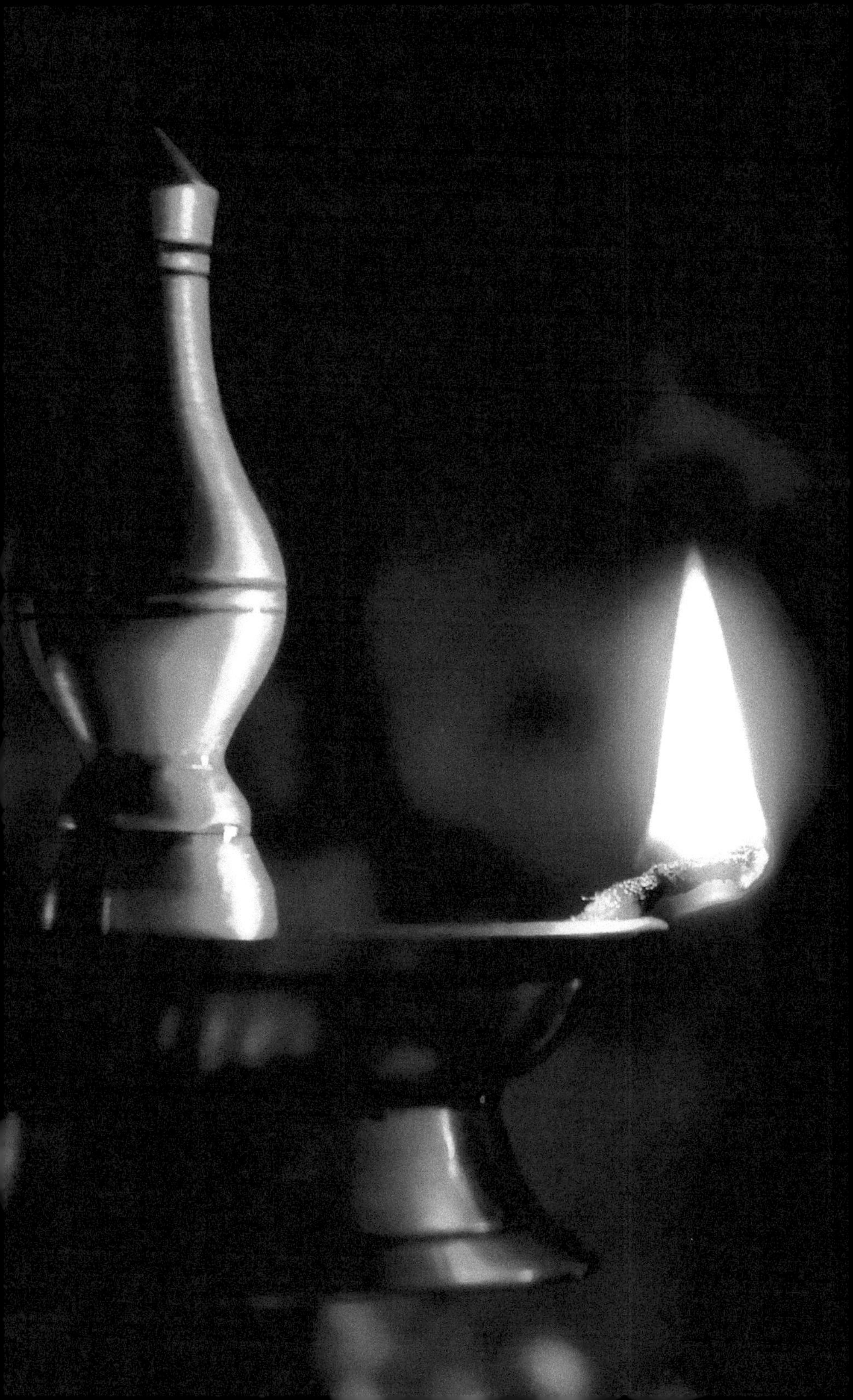

pranayamas have an excellent effect on strong overheating, irritation and emotions.

KAPHA

Breathing through the right nostril is well suited for the morning as it reduces kapha. Bhastrika and kapalbhati are excellent for kaphas, especially for countering the effects of colds (not fever), listlessness and depression.

MEDITATION

Meditation consists mainly of dharana (concentration), dhyana (meditation), and samadhi (ecstasy). These three steps belong to the inner aspect of the eight steps of yoga. In Ayurveda, meditation is used for therapeutic purposes, mainly to heal the mind and psychological diseases. Still, its effect also affects our physical body as our physical body is also affected by our mental state. The body, prana, and senses must be balanced to meditate.

Both the body and the mind are made up of the five elements. The body comprises elements heavy in character, such as earth and water (kapha), which shape our body. The body's functions consist of slightly lighter elements and doshas. Pitta (fire) is responsible for bodily transformations, while vata (air) is responsible for the impulses between our brain and nerve impulses. The mind is made up of the lighter form of vata (air and ether), which makes it volatile. The mind's functions consist of the heavier elements: fire, water, and earth (pitta and kapha). Fire gives the mind perceptions, the water adds emotions, and the earth connects the mind with the body. The mind is fast and in perpetual change.

Vatas are more quick-witted than other dosha types. It is easier for them to make new acquaintances (air) and be open to new experiences (ether). Vatas have very active senses and are always on the move somewhere. They are more often affected by mental and psychological imbalances.

Pitta is seen as the insightful part of the mind, with the third eye of the mind relating to the element of fire. The fire of reason is called buddhi (intellect and insight). Pitta types are often brilliant, with an excellent ability to focus and have sharp and clear thinking.

Kaphas feel emotions, love, and devotion linked to our senses and the external character of the mind (manas). Bliss, as the core of the mind, is the highest form of kapha.

Meditation allows us to come in contact with our higher self and consciousness (atman and purusha). With the help of meditation, we can cleanse our subconscious from things that cause us suffering. Regardless of the meditation technique used, the purpose is to create the original stillness of our consciousness, which is our true nature.

Meditation can help with:
– Psychological diseases.
– Difficulty falling asleep.
– Emotional disorders.
– Chronic diseases such as allergies and asthma that are affected by stress and hypersensitivity in the nervous system.
– Heart disease. According to ancient Vedic texts, our consciousness belongs to the heart. Therefore, calming the mind and strengthening the heart go hand in hand.
– Pain relief by, e.g., focusing on a mantra.
– Preparing for death and leaving the body.

MEDITATION FOR VATA

Meditation can help vatas with their hypersensitive and active mind to provide better sleep, improve metabolism, and strengthen the immune system. Caution must be exercised as meditation performed incorrectly can have the opposite effect on vatas and cause feelings of volatility. Vatas should first and foremost exercise their ability to concentrate. Techniques that include mantras and visualization are good because they saturate the mind instead of "emptying" it. Vatas should not try to calm the natural flow of thoughts but observe and let it flow.

Preparation:
– Relaxing asanas help vata types sit for more extended periods.

– Deep breathing exercises increase concentration by providing the body with prana.

Visualizations:
– Earth, fire, and water.
– Mountains, lakes, flowers, fire, and sunset.

Balancing colors:
– Gold and saffron help vata types achieve mental clarity.

Mantras:
– Ram, Shrim, and Hrim.
During meditation or when vata seems to be out of balance.

Deities to meditate on:
– Durga and Tara give a feeling of security.
– Shiva and Vishnu give a feeling of security.
– Ganesha creates a sense of grounding.

Considering vata's anxious and fearful nature, devotion to a god or any teacher or guru is suitable. In this way, vatas can leave their worries and problems to someone else, get help, and experience security at the same time.

Vatas must learn to experience contact with the eternal within itself, create stability, and not worry about the changing world. Vatas need space and peace to escape the pace of their surroundings. Meditation on the true eternal helps to slow down one's thoughts.

MEDITATION FOR PITTA

Pitta people need meditation to release emotions such as aggression and anger. They often have an excellent ability to concentrate, and it is easy for them to meditate. Mantra meditation is a perfect way for pittas to maximize their solid mental energy by focusing it on a goal. Pitta types must work to expand their mind and heart with the help of the inner light and thus gain insight into the truth. The meditation should provide stillness in the mind and heart of the pitta.

Preparation:
- Soothing asanas that do not create too much heat in the body.
- Shitali pranayama, or breathing through the left nostril to cool the system.

Visualizations:
- Mountains, forests, lakes, and seas.
- Rain clouds, flowers in cold colors, the moon and the stars.

Balancing colors:
- White, dark blue, and green.

Affirmations:
– Devotion, love, and forgiveness to balance the fire.
– Prayers for peace and love for other people.

Mantras:
– Shrim, Sham, and Om. Recited silently.

Deities to meditate on:
– Lakshmi, Uma Parvati, Shiva, and Vishnu.

Pittas can be very critical and judgmental. They can use and transform this power by redirecting it to explore their inner self and expand their consciousness. Meditating on infinite space beyond all limitations is beneficial to their critical minds.

MEDITATION FOR KAPHA

Kaphas need meditation to free themselves from old emotional and mental patterns and to counteract inertia. Kaphas need a lot of encouragement and motivation to meditate, so group meditation is usually best suited for them.

It is easy for kaphas to fall asleep and daydream, so choosing an active form of meditation can help prevent this from happening. A combined form of meditation and activity with mantras or pranayamas is good.

Preparation:
– Powerful asanas that start the circulation in the body.
– Bhastrika pranayama, or breathing through the right nostril.

Visualization:
– Fire, air, and ether.
– Sun, wind, sky.

Balancing colors:
– Gold, blue, and orange.

Affirmations:
– Which strengthens the connection to the higher self.
For example. "In my true self, I am independent and free, in nature and space."

Mantras:
– Om, Hum and Aim.
Cleansing and stimulating, to be recited out loud.

Deities to meditate on:
– Shiva and Kali. Divinities of an angry nature release emotions and reduce the ego.

Meditating on emptiness and the inner light creates more space and fire in the mind, which benefits kaphas.

PULSE DIAGNOSTICS

In Ayurveda, various techniques are used to establish a diagnosis of one's health. These include analysis of heart rate, urine, feces, eyes, tongue, speech, skin, shape, and most importantly, pulse. Taking one's pulse as a diagnostic tool has been used in Ayurveda since immemorial. A well-experienced Ayurvedic physicist can use the pulse to assess prakruti (one's general constitution), vikruti (current imbalances in the doshas), subtle imbalances, and other diseases.

You can read the pulse in different places in the body – e.g., in the armpit, ankle, and wrist, of which the latter is the most common. It is done by placing the index finger, middle finger, and ring finger on the upper side of the wrist (towards the thumb). The three fingers represent the different doshas: vata, pitta, and kapha. The index finger represents the vata dosha, the middle finger represents the pitta dosha, and the ring finger represents the kapha dosha. Each dosha has a characteristic pulse: from where the pulse starts, where on the finger it beats the strongest, from which direction it hits, and what quality the pulse has. Rishis use animal movement patterns to describe heart rate levels:

The vata pulse's movement pattern can be compared to how a cobra moves. It is fast, weak, cold, thin, disappears with pressure, and is best felt under the index finger.

The pitta pulse's movement pattern can be compared to a frog. It is prominent, robust, warm, and influential, lifts the palpating finger, and best feels under the middle finger.

The kapha pulse's movement can be likened to a swimming swan. It is deep, slow, wide, wavy, dense, cold or hot, regular, and can be best felt under the ring finger.

THE SEVEN LEVELS OF THE PULSE

In Ayurveda, the pulse is divided into seven levels, each of which tells us how we feel mentally, physically, and spiritually. You can read the different levels by placing three palpating fingers on the wrist and changing the pressure. The pulses provide the practitioner with vikruti (imbalances) in our doshas. Manas vikruti (manas: mind).

SUBDOSHA

Each dosha(vata, pitta, and kapha) has five subdoshas. Each sub dosha represents a particular aspect of our physiology. In each sub dosha, one of the five elements is prominent.

Vata subdoshas: prana, udana, samana, vyana and apana.

Pitta subdoshas: pachaka, ranjaka, alochaka, sadhaka and bharajaka.

Kapha subdoshas: kledaka, avalambaka, bodhaka, tarpaka and shleshaka.

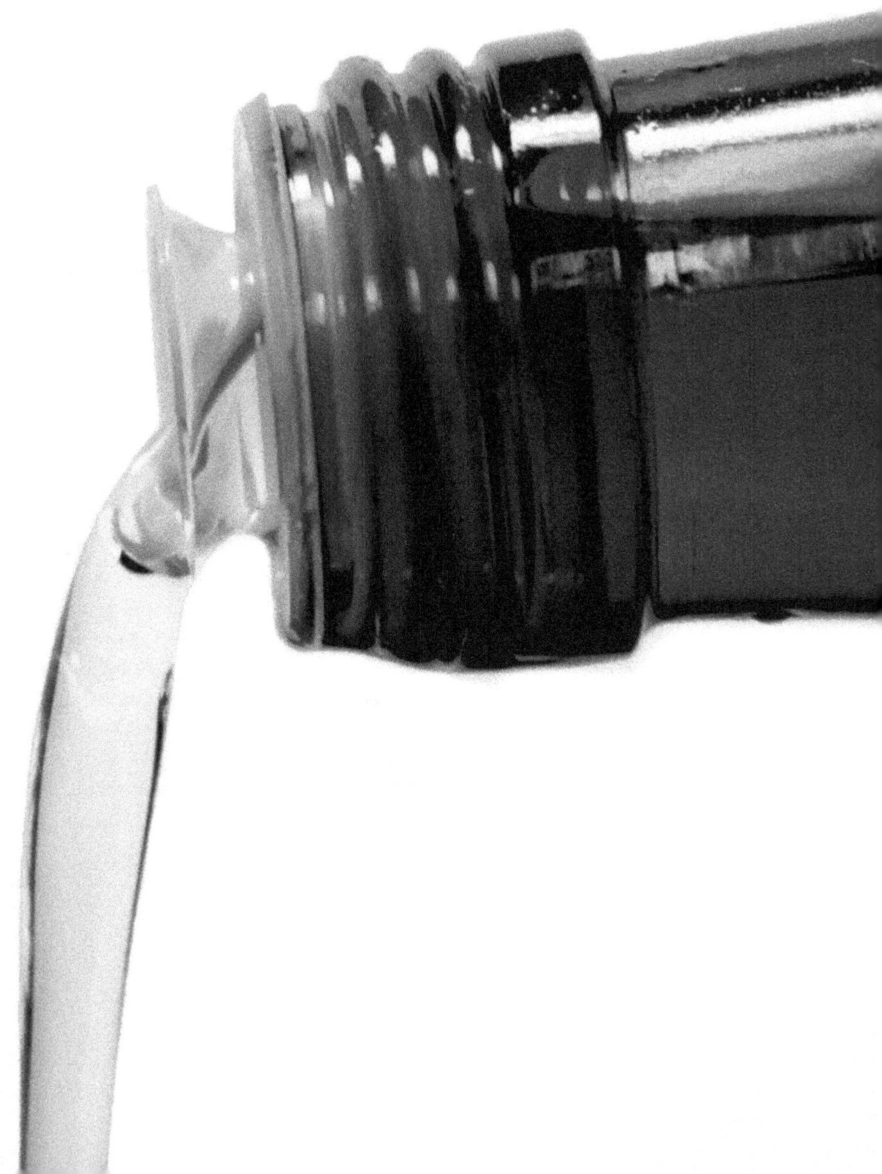

Prana, tejas and ojas. Prana is the essence of vata, tejas is the essence of pitta, and ojas is the essence of kapha. Ojas are created during nutrition and are the main essence of all tissues. Tejas can be compared to hormones and amino acids. Prana, which is the vital life energy, is responsible for the cooperation between cells.

Dhatus represents our biological tissues, such as plasma, blood, muscle, fat, bones, nerves, and male and female reproductive tissues.

Prakruti represents our basic psychosomatic and biological constitution. Manas Prakruti (manas: sun). If a person says they are, for example, a pitta person, they are not talking about any imbalance but their essential constitution.

CHINESE MEDICINE

Pulse diagnostics is also an essential part of Chinese medicine. However, Ayurvedic pulse diagnostics and Chinese differ somewhat. In Chinese technology, one can read forty-seven aspects of the pulse, compared with the seven levels in Ayurveda.

AYURVEDIC TREATMENTS

In Ayurvedic treatment, there are eight main disciplines, so-called ashtangas:

Internal medicine (kaya-chikitsa).

Pediatrics (kaumarabhrityam).

Surgery (shalya-chikitsa).

Eyes (shalakya-tantra).

The science of demonic obsession (bhuta-vidya). It has been called psychiatry.

Toxicology (agada-tantram).

Disease prevention, immunity enhancement, and rejuvenation (rasayana).

Aphrodisiacs and improving the health of the offspring (vaji-karanam).

AYURVEDIC MASSAGE

Ayurvedic massage is used to treat various diseases and for preventive purposes.

There are at least forty different types of Ayurvedic massage, which, along with various other diagnostic tools, are used by Ayurvedic doctors to treat diseases and ill health.

Ayurvedic massage relieves pain, relaxes stiff muscles, reduces swelling caused by joint inflammation, improves blood circulation, increases stress resistance, provides better sleep, increases athletic performance, and provides emotional benefits. With Ayurvedic massage, deeply rooted toxins are released in joints and tissues and eliminated through natural processes.

ABHYANGA – AYURVEDIC OIL MASSAGE

Abhyanga (oil massage) is a standard Ayurvedic massage. Abhyanga is a therapeutic massage of about forty-five minutes and is used to treat many diseases. Two therapists working on the client's side often give Abhyanga, lying on a wooden bed. Particular attention is paid to the feet because there are marma points (nerve nodes) on the soles of the feet that are closely related to specific internal organs. The sole of the right foot is massaged clockwise, and the left is counter-clockwise.

During treatment, the client rests in seven standard positions. Abhyanga begins with the client sitting in an upright position, after which she lies flat on her back, turns to the right side, lies on her back again, turns to the left side, lies on her back again, and finally returns to a sitting position. Abhyanga is an essential part of pancha karma therapy.

SHIRO ABHYANGA – AYURVEDIC HEAD MASSAGE

Shiro abhyanga is a head massage with roots in Ayurveda. The purpose of Shiro abhyanga is not only to ward off stress but also to stimulate the body to heal itself. Various oils are usually included as a natural part of the treatment to soothe the soul and care for the skin and hair. Shiro abhyanga is a head massage that, in addition to Ayurvedic contexts, is common in hair salons in India.

NASYAM – AYURVEDIC NASAL TREATMENT

Nasyam is an Ayurvedic treatment in which medicinal oils are administered through the nose to clear the throat, nose, and head of harmful substances.

This treatment is used to treat migraines, headaches, mental disorders, prematurely graying hair, and speech difficulties. Nasyam is also said to strengthen the mind and intellect and is included in pancha karma treatment.

PANCHA KARMA

The most famous form of Ayurvedic treatment is pancha karma. Pancha karma, or literally "five actions" in Sanskrit, is a cleansing treatment to increase the metabolic process with an appropriate diet, natural herbs, and minerals. Pancha karma is used for deep-rooted chronic diseases and seasonal imbalances of the three elemental energies (doshas): pitta, vata, and kapha. The treatment aims to make the body healthy by eliminating bodily waste products and achieving a balance between the doshas.

Pancha karma – five actions in three steps.

The five measures consist of nasyan (nasal treatment), vamana (vomiting), virechana (detoxing), nirooha vasti (enemas with herbal decoctions), and sneha vasti (enemas with herbal oils). After these treatments, hopefully, the body has been cleansed of accumulated toxins.

Panchakarma is always performed in three stages: purva karma (pre-treatment), pradhana karma (primary treatment) and paschat karma (post-treatment). The patient who chooses any of the five treatments above must always undergo all three stages for the treatment to have the intended effect.

Step 1. Pre-treatment (purva karma).
Snehana (oil therapy) is an essential preparatory treatment. Snehana is said to loosen toxins stuck in different places in the body and is often given with adapted herbal mixtures to treat an individual disease. Still, it can also be provided in a pure form without additives. Snehana is given early in the morning for a maximum of seven days and is said to help transfer toxins to the gastrointestinal tract so that they can be easily removed afterward. If snehana is not given before pancha karma, the intended effect on the treatment will not be obtained.

Oil massage (abhyanga) is another crucial treatment in pancha karma.

Svedana is a therapy that induces sweating and is administered to the whole body or parts of the body, depending on the disease. Steam with added medicinal herbs is usually used, but it can also be achieved by having the patient sit under the sun while thirsty and hungry, covering their body with thick sheets, or staying in a closed, dark room. Svedana is said to dilate ducts in the body and thus helps move toxins to the gastrointestinal tract.

Step 2. Primary treatment (pradhana karma).
The toxins and slag products that reach the gastrointestinal tract are believed to be eliminated during the primary treatment.

One of the five primary treatments, vamana karma, is used for kapha diseases such as bronchitis, colds, coughs, asthma, sinusitis, and excess mucus. One to three days before vamana karma, one is treated with oil internally and externally through abhyanga (Ayurvedic massage) and internally with ghee (shredded butter) in the diet.

Step 3. Post-treatment (paschat karma).
The finishing treatment consists of adapted diets, appropriate physical effort, and intake of herbs to promote long-term health.

AYURVEDA AND SESAME OIL

Sesame oil is extracted from sesame seeds and is often used in cooking as a seasoning, but in Ayurveda, it is also used for massage and skin care. It has been used for thousands of years in India due to its healing effects.

In Ayurveda, regular massage with sesame oil is recommended to achieve many health benefits. Ayurveda practitioners believe that massage with sesame oil cleanses, balances the lymphatic and endocrine systems, lubricates, and softens muscles, tissues, and joints. They also think that the oil makes the skin radiant and youthful. Sesame oil is the best oil to use due to its ability to penetrate the skin and because it is generally recommended for all body constitutions, whether you are a vata, kapha, or pitta.

According to Ayurveda, sesame oil is excellent because it is naturally antibacterial against common skin pathogens, such as staphylococci and streptococci, and common skin fungi, such as athlete's foot. It is also naturally antiviral and anti-inflammatory.

Additionally, sesame oil is considered to relieve or cure psoriasis, dry scalp, irritated skin, and skin rashes in teens, regulate pore enlargement, and heal or protect wounds.

AYURVEDIC MASSAGE IN THE HOME

How to do Ayurvedic oil massage at home.

1. Before starting the massage, warm the oil to body temperature or higher. Start by massaging your head. Dip your fingertips into the oil and massage the oil into the scalp. During the entire massage, use as much of the whole palm of your hand as possible, not just the fingertips. Since the head is one of the most essential body parts to massage, feel free to spend more time there than the other parts.

2. Gently lubricate the face and outer ears—massage with the entire palm where possible. Massage your face and neck gently. Do not massage as firmly here as on other body parts.

3. Then massage the neck and upper spine with open hands and light movements.

4. It is good to apply the oil on all body parts and then start again from the top and massage. This way, the oil has time to stay on the skin longer.

5. Continue with your arms. Massage with reciprocating movements (long up and down movements) along the long muscles and circulating movements over the joints.

6. Proceed to the chest and abdomen—massage over the

heart with light circular motions. Massage the abdomen clockwise from the lower right side upwards to the more down left side.

7. Massage all parts of the back and spine as far as you can.

8. Continue with the legs—massage with reciprocating movements along the large muscles and circulating movements over the joints.

9. Finally, massage your feet. Like the head, the feet are considered one of the most essential body parts to rub. Please spend a little more time here. Massage the soles of the feet with the entire palm.

10. Finish with a hot bath or shower.

Did you like the book? Feel free to follow me on my social media, share and like, tell your friends about the books, and feel free to write an honest review; one or two lines don't matter. All support is precious. Thanks!

On my Facebook page and Instagram, I post exciting news and tips on temporary offers and benefits you can take advantage of. I often also post my yoga routine and other things related to nutrition and health that may be interesting to take part in. So feel free to join them so you don't miss anything interesting:

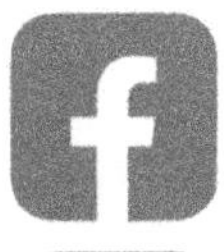 *facebook.com/bhagwanoneofakindbooks*

 *instagram.com/bhagwanoneofakindbooks/*

MY BOOKS AND BOOK SERIES

I have two book series that have different audiences. Great Yoga Books – is a series with the most comprehensive fact books on yoga for those who want to explore the subject in depth. Here, you will also find classic yoga books that are rarely translated, such as Patanjali's Yoga Sutras and Hatha Yoga Pradipika. My second series, Yoga Beyond the Poses: The Ultimate Beginner's Guide to Yoga, covers one yoga topic at a time and is extra easy to read with larger text. For those who find it challenging to read extensive books and want a good and broad overview of the subject quickly. Both series are also available as audiobooks.

★★★★★

TEACHING YOGA
&
MEDITATION
BEYOND
THE POSES

BESTSELLING AUTHOR

Shreyananda Natha

Teaching Yoga and Meditation Beyond the Poses – A unique and practical workbook!

Teaching Yoga and Meditation Beyond the Poses – A unique and practical workbook for aspiring yoga teachers who want to teach yoga and meditation beyond the poses.

Teaching Yoga and Meditation Beyond the Poses is a unique and essential resource for new and experienced teachers and a guide for all yoga students interested in refining their skills and knowledge. Teaching Yoga and Meditation is also ideal as a core textbook in yoga teacher training programs.

The book covers fundamental yoga philosophy and history topics, including a historical presentation of classical yoga literature: Yoga Sutras of Patanjali, Bhagavad Gita, etc. Each of the seven major styles of yoga is described, from Hatha yoga, Raja yoga, Tantra yoga, Bhakti yoga, and Kundalini yoga, to knowledge about the chakras, Ayurveda and magic mantras and yantras. The book provides extensive support and tools for teaching integrated and classical yoga (asanas), breathing techniques (pranayama), deep relaxation (Yoga Nidra), and meditation (Ajapa Japa). The book is divided into eight modules with associated knowledge tests and complete yoga and meditation classes.

https://rb.gy/9s6edj

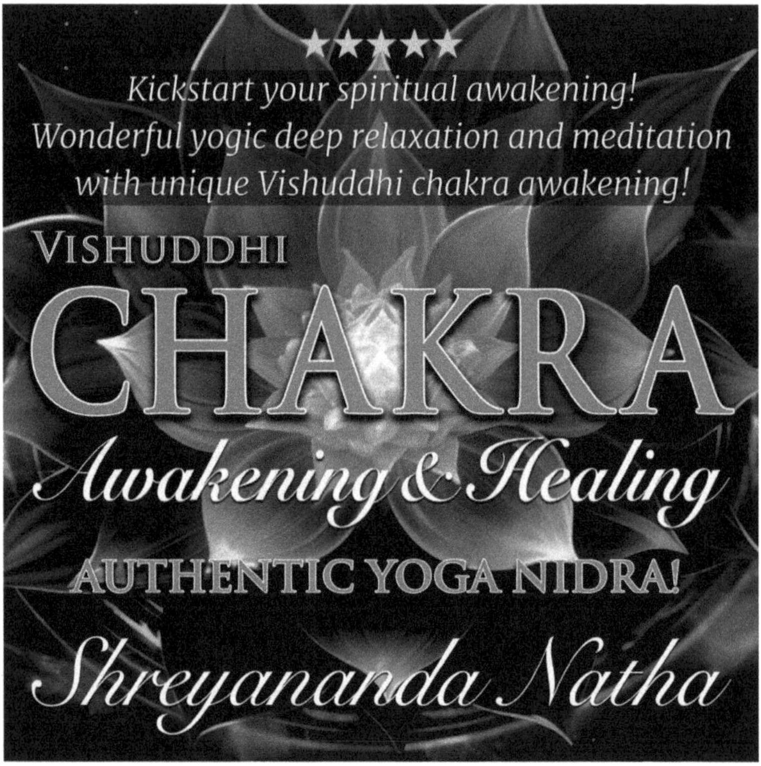

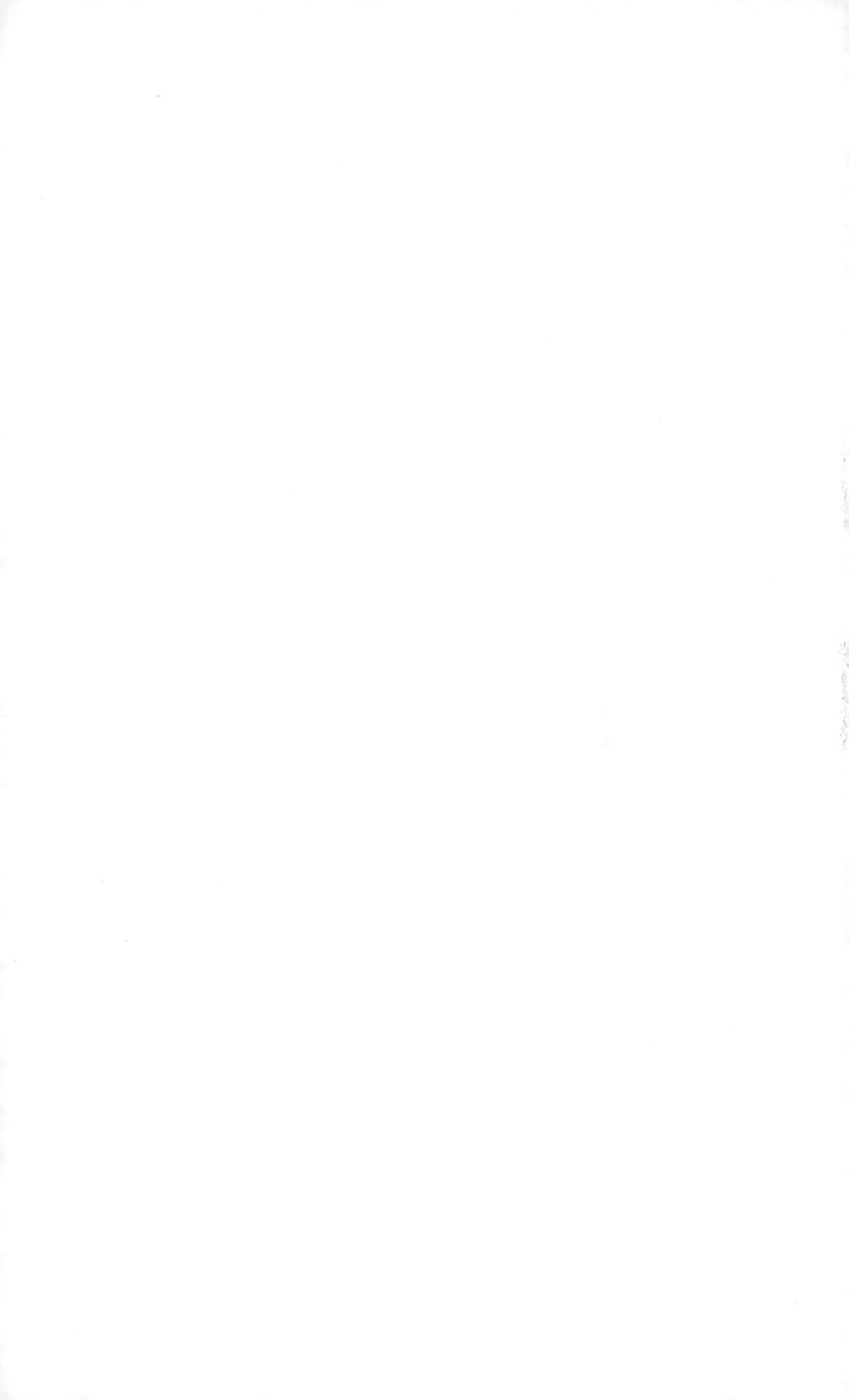